Pride and Pollution

Pride and Pollution

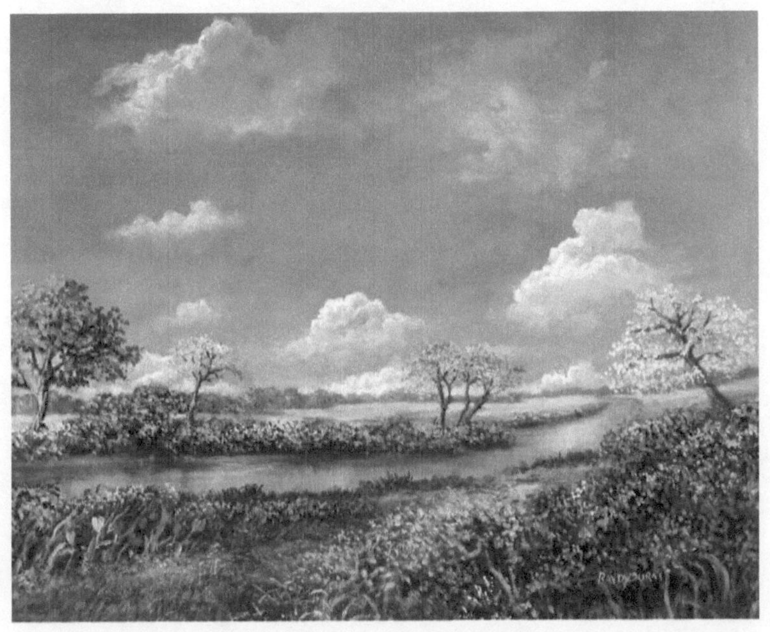

Gene Allen Groner

In Honor of the Wonderful

World Created by God.

"There is only one God, the father of us all who created everything that exists."_Apostle Paul

To

From

Copyright © 2020 by Gene Allen Groner

Bible translations are from the New King James Version (NKJV) unless otherwise indicated.

Introduction

I wrote Pride and Pollution in an effort to encourage more people around the world to become active agents of change.

God created a wonderful and beautiful world—a world filled with trees, birds, blue skies, clean seas, and all manner of wildlife—healthy and happy and thriving.

The desire of my heart is to give my grandchildren and their children the world as God intended it to be.

To that end, I present this book as an offering to God.

I pray in Jesus' wonderful name, amen.

Chapter One

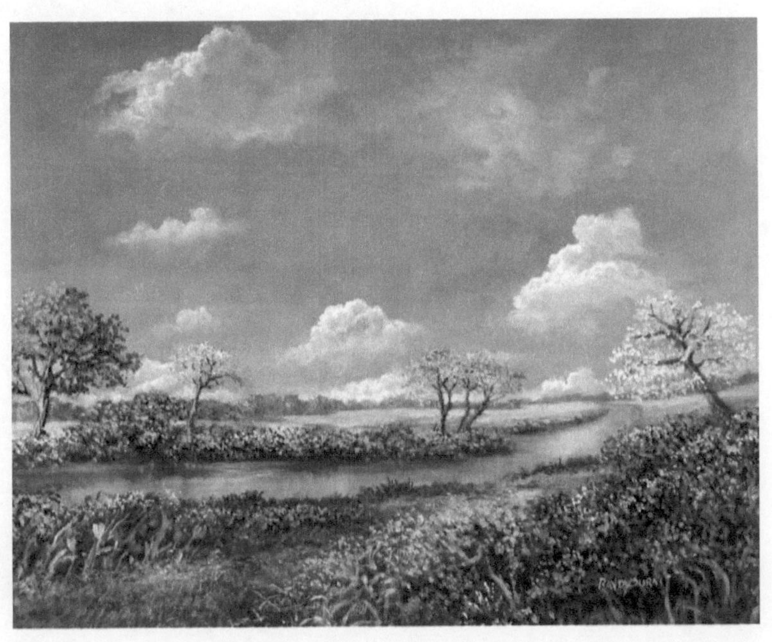

In the Beginning

"The top environmental problems are selfishness, greed, and apathy. To deal with these we need a cultural and spiritual transformation."

—Gus Speth, former dean of the Yale School of Forestry and Environmental Studies, founder and president of the World Resources Institute.

"A cultural and spiritual transformation."

"Almost a half century has flown by since we launched the Natural Resources Defense Council. Over that period NRDC and other mainstream U.S. environmental groups have racked up more victories and accomplishments than we can count. One shudders to think what our world would be like had they not.

Yet, despite those accomplishments, a specter is haunting American environmentalism—the specter of failure. All of us who have been part of the environmental movement in the United States must now face up to a deeply troubling paradox: Our environmental organizations have grown in strength and sophistication, but the environment has continued to go downhill.

The prospect of a ruined planet is now very real. We have won many victories, but we are losing the planet." (from James Gustave Speth's Angels by the River).

I have grown increasingly concerned about the earth we live in, the air we breathe, the food we eat, and the rapidly growing pollution of the earth's seas and lakes and rivers.

The forests of the Amazon provide most of the medicine for the planet, and they are being decimated by the industrialization of corporate greed, and by the pollution caused by climate change and poisonous chemicals and gases.

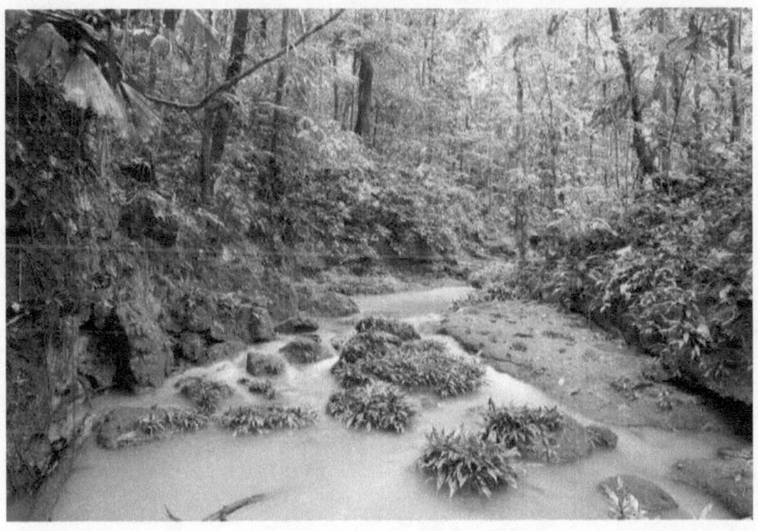

A Stream in the Amazon Rainforest in Ecuador

The Amazon Rainforest in South America covers 6,000,000 square kilometers (2.3 million square miles) and several million species of insects, plants, birds, and other forms of life, some of the richest on earth.

However, life there is rapidly dying due to cutting, burning, farming, and grazing. The borders of the forest are being pushed back by humanity's negligence and lack of concern for one of the richest ecological systems on earth.

"Some 75,000 fires occurred in the Brazilian Amazon during the first half of 2019 (an increase of 85 percent over 2018), largely due to encouragement from Brazilian Pres. Jair Bolsonaro, a strong proponent of tree clearing." (source: Encyclopedia Britannica)

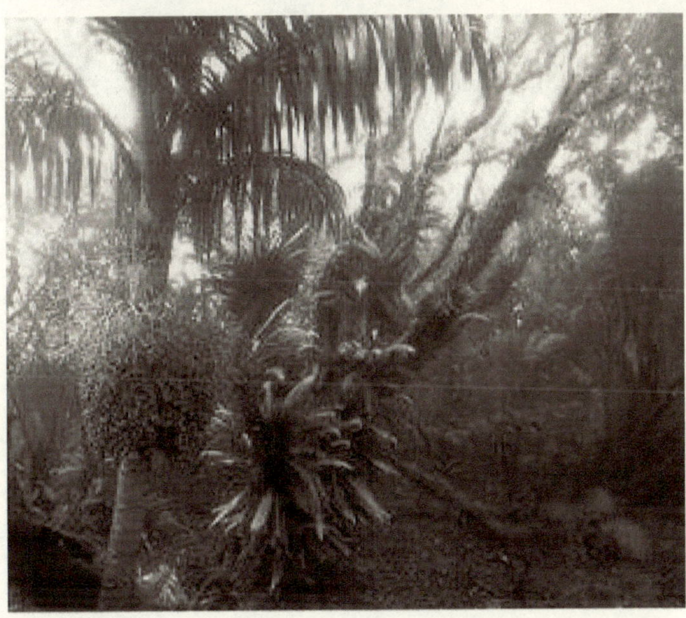

1 <u>In the beginning</u> God created the heavens and the earth. 2 The earth was without form, and void; and darkness was on the face of the deep. And the Spirit of God was hovering over the face of the waters.

3 Then God said, "Let there be light"; and there was light. 4 And God saw the light, that it was good; and God divided the light from the darkness. 5 God called the light Day, and the darkness He called Night. So the evening and the morning were the first day.

6 Then God said, "Let there be a firmament in the midst of the waters, and let it divide the waters from the waters." 7 Thus God made the firmament, and divided the waters which were under the firmament from the waters which were above the firmament; and it was so. 8 And God called the firmament Heaven. So the evening and the morning were the second day.

9 Then God said, "Let the waters under the heavens be gathered together into one place, and let the dry land appear"; and it was so. 10 And God called the dry land Earth, and the gathering together of the waters He called Seas. And God saw that it was good.

11 Then God said, "Let the earth bring forth grass, the herb that yields seed, and the fruit tree that yields fruit according to its kind, whose seed is in itself, on the earth"; and it was so. 12 And the earth brought forth grass, the herb that yields seed according to its kind, and the tree that yields fruit, whose seed is in itself according to its kind. And God saw that it was good. 13 So the evening and the morning were the third day.

14 Then God said, "Let there be lights in the firmament of the heavens to divide the day from the night; and let them be for signs and seasons, and for days and years; 15 and let them be for lights in the firmament of the heavens to give light on the earth"; and it was so. 16 Then God made two great lights: the greater light to rule the day, and the lesser light to rule the night. He made the stars also. 17 God set them in the firmament of the heavens to give light on the earth, 18 and to rule over the day and over the night, and to divide the light from the darkness. And God saw that it was good. 19 So the evening and the morning were the fourth day.

20 Then God said, "Let the waters abound with an abundance of living creatures, and let birds fly above the earth across the face of the

firmament of the heavens." 21 So God created great sea creatures and every living thing that moves, with which the waters abounded, according to their kind, and every winged bird according to its kind. And God saw that it was good. 22 And God blessed them, saying, "Be fruitful and multiply, and fill the waters in the seas, and let birds multiply on the earth." 23 So the evening and the morning were the fifth day. (Genesis 1 NJKV)

<u>In the beginning,</u> God created a wonderful and beautiful world for us, and commanded us to care for it so that it would always provide our needs. When God said to "subdue" the world, he was asking us to be good stewards, and use the things of this world for our good, not for our greed. Stewards take good care of things.

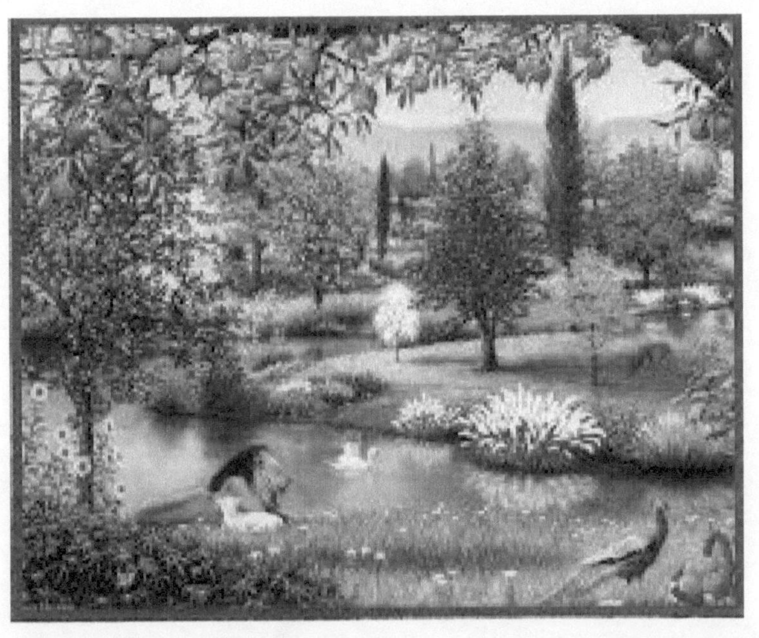

Chapter Two

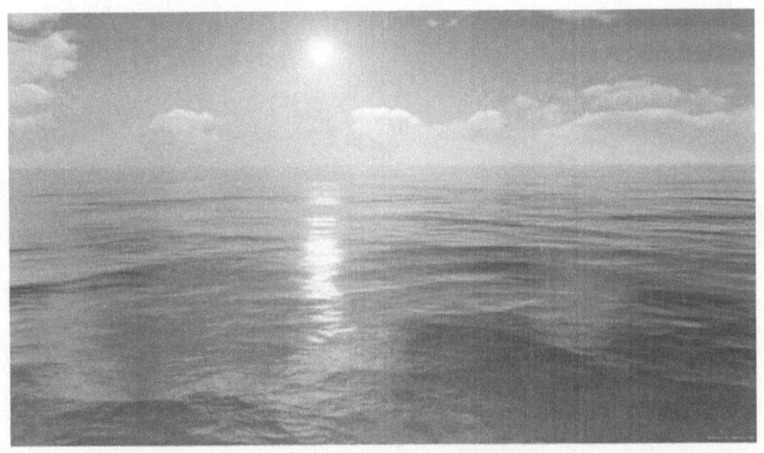

Oceans of the World

I've been privileged to travel over many of the world's oceans, seas, lakes and rivers—the Atlantic Ocean, Pacific Ocean, Mediterranean Sea, Gulf of Mexico, the Caribbean, The St. Lawrence River of Canada, the Jordan River in Israel, and many others.

Clean water and good sanitation is a blessing.

The World Health Organization states that 2 billion people in the world do not have safe water for drinking because it's contaminated with feces, and an estimated 2.5 billion people do not have safe sanitation to prevent disease and death.

That is unconscionable, considering God has created enough clean water for everyone on earth.

485,000 people die every year from diarrhea caused by contaminated water.

"Safe and readily available water is important for public health, whether it is used for drinking, domestic use, food production or recreational purposes. Improved water supply and sanitation, and better management of water resources, can boost countries' economic growth and can contribute greatly to poverty reduction.

In 2010, the UN General Assembly explicitly recognized the human right to water and sanitation. Everyone has the right to sufficient, continuous, safe, acceptable, physically accessible, and affordable water for personal and domestic use." (source: the World Health Organization in 2019)

I pray every day for those who do not have these blessings of life. But prayer alone will not solve the problem. It takes action. It takes those who are willing to be agents of positive change in the world. It takes you and me to make a difference.

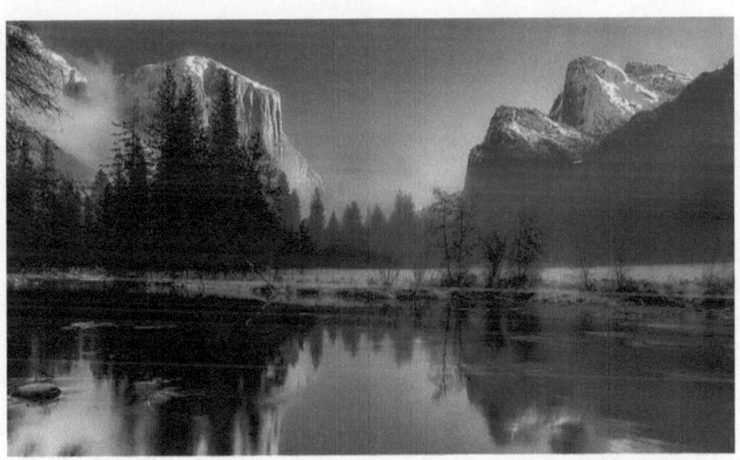

Chapter Three

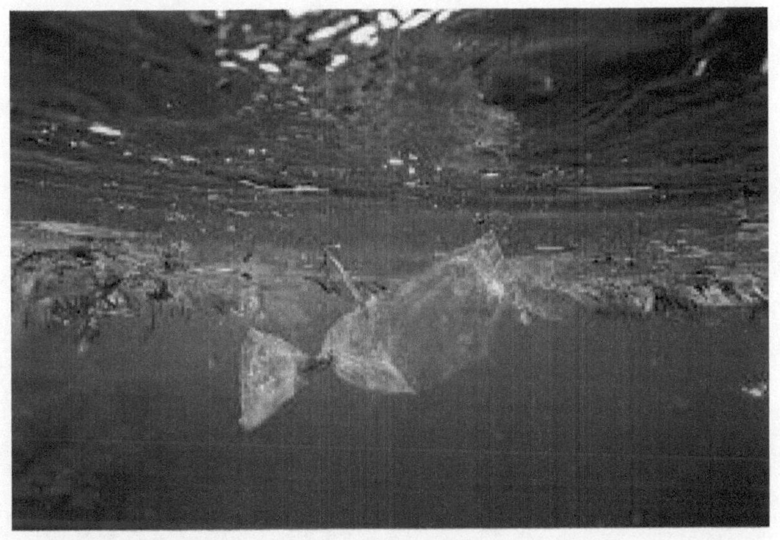

Ocean and River Pollution

"Rivers are the main source of ocean plastic pollution. They are the arteries that carry waste from land to the ocean. Our research found that 1000 rivers are responsible for roughly 80% of the pollution.

To rid the oceans of plastic, we need to not only clean up what is already out there, but also stop new plastic from entering the ocean: we need to close the tap."

(source: OceanCleanup.com)

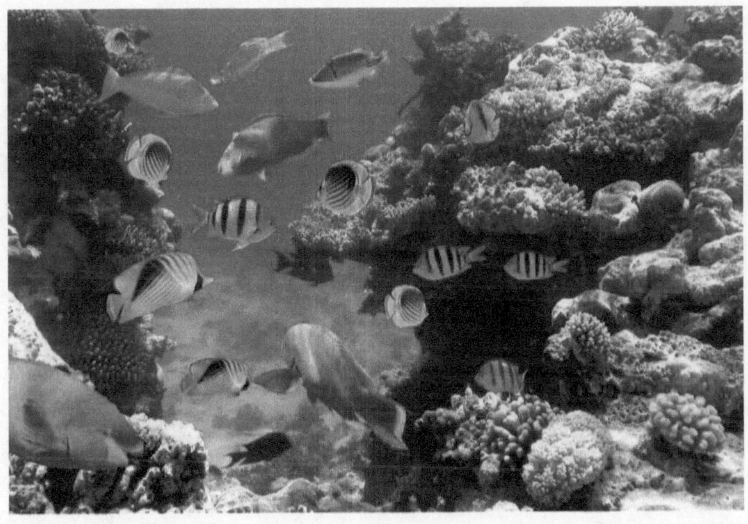

The ocean is a beautiful thing to behold. I have enjoyed my time swimming and snorkeling in

the seas, and sailing in Kaneohe Bay in Hawaii.
I never get tired of watching the wildlife in the
documentaries of National Geographic on
television. I don't want to lose this beauty, and
I hope my grandchildren will be able to say the
same thing about our oceans and seas and
lakes and rivers—valuable resources given to
us by God. We are the stewards over it all.

As I think about our oceans and lakes and
rivers, I am reminded of something I wrote a
while back. It is a short story about Jesus and
the Woman at the Well.

Let me tell you about it. It's called Living
Water.

Living Water

"The water that I will give will become a well of
water springing up to eternal life."

These are the words of Jesus that he spoke to
the woman of Samaria that warm summer day.
She was thirsty. He gave her water to drink.
She was tired. He offered her rest for her soul.
She was weary of the life she had lived. He
gave her a new life and a new hope for the
future.

She had many husbands. Jesus told her she only needed one. He was the one she needed.

Jesus is the one we need.

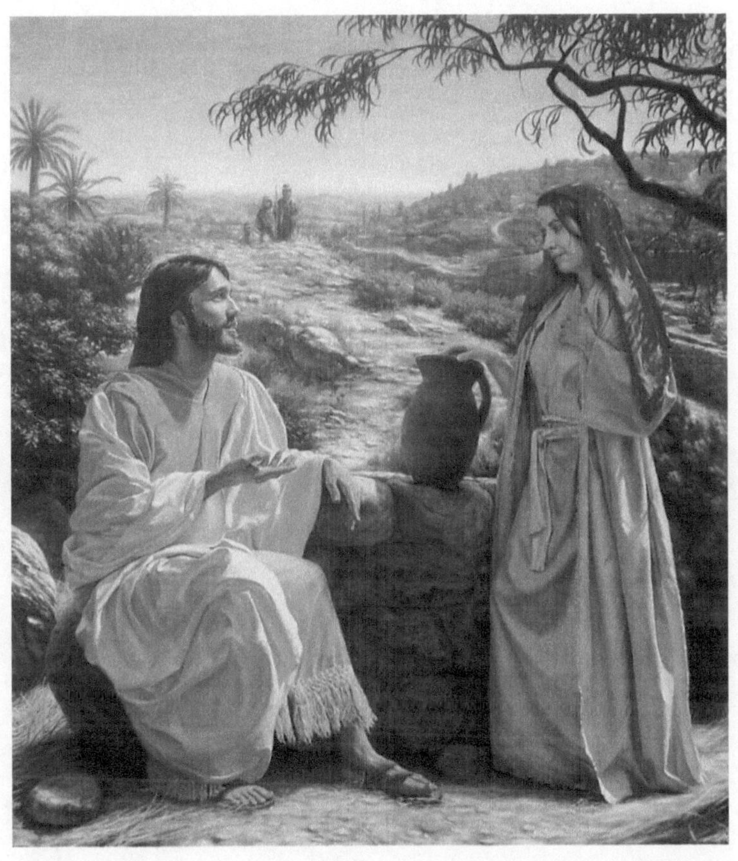

Jesus and the Woman at the Well—John 4:1-42

Behind my house is a living spring. Every day it brings forth fresh water from the earth.

It never fails, never falters, it never forgets. Fresh water every day without missing a drop.

When I think of the water from our living spring, it reminds me of Jesus and his everlasting love, the kind of love I need. I am no different than the woman from Samaria.

We are the same, she and I. We both drink from the same well, the well touched by the hands of Jesus.

The same hands that healed the blind and the lame. The same hands that blessed the bread and the wine. The same hands that prayed to the Father. The same hands that blessed the little children; that lifted the fearful and drowning Peter up from the Sea. The same hands that raised Lazarus from the dead.

Hands that will never grow old or tired. Hands that are made for touching and holding and blessing.

Hands that are full of love for the poor. Hands reaching out to heal and to bless and to forgive.

How I love those hands. Those are the hands that I long to touch. Those are the hands that we all want to hold. Those are the hands that created the world. Those are the hands that heal the broken-hearted.

One day those same hands will take us home.

Home to the place where we belong.

Home to the place of light and love.

Home to the place where God the Father waits for us.

 Home to the place of living water.

That's my home. Heaven.

Chapter Four

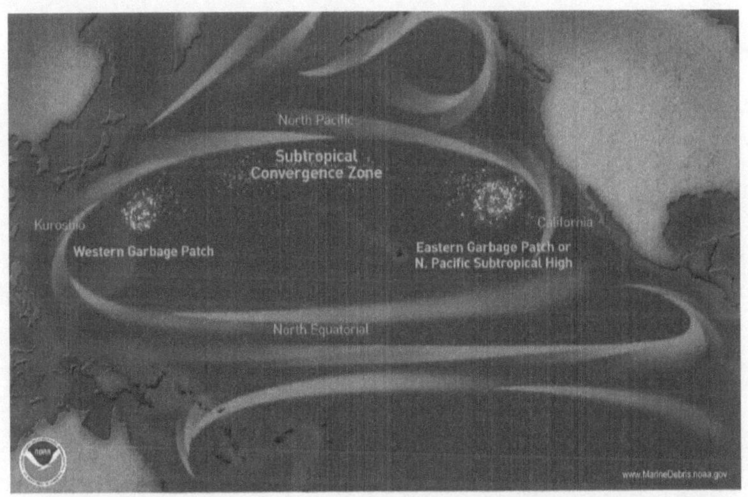

Pollution in the Pacific

National Geographic reports, "The Great Pacific Garbage Patch, also known as the Pacific trash vortex, spans waters from the West Coast of North America to Japan. The patch is actually composed of the Western Garbage Patch, located near Japan, and the Eastern Garbage Patch, located between the U.S. states of Hawaii and California.

These areas of spinning debris are linked together by the North Pacific Subtropical Convergence Zone, located a few hundred kilometers north of Hawaii. This convergence zone is where warm water from the South Pacific meets up with cooler water from the Arctic. The zone acts like a highway that moves debris from one patch to another.

The entire Great Pacific Garbage Patch is bounded by the North Pacific Subtropical Gyre. The National Oceanic and Atmospheric Administration (NOAA) defines a gyre as a large system of swirling ocean currents. Increasingly, however, it also refers to the garbage patch / a vortex of plastic waste and debris broken down into small particles in the ocean. The North Pacific Subtropical Gyre is formed by four currents rotating clockwise around an area of 20 million square kilometers (7.7 million square miles): the California

"current, the North Equatorial current, the Kuroshio current, and the North Pacific current.

The area in the center of a gyre tends to be very calm and stable. The circular motion of the gyre draws debris into this stable center, where it becomes trapped. A plastic water bottle discarded off the coast of California, for instance, takes the California Current south toward Mexico. There, it may catch the North Equatorial Current, which crosses the vast Pacific. Near the coast of Japan, the bottle may travel north on the powerful Kuroshio Current. Finally, the bottle travels westward on the North Pacific Current. The gently rolling vortexes of the Eastern and Western Garbage Patches gradually draw in the bottle.

The amount of debris in the Great Pacific Garbage Patch accumulates because much of it is not biodegradable. Many plastics, for instance, do not wear down; they simply break into tinier and tinier pieces.

For many people, the idea of a "garbage patch" conjures up images of an island of trash floating on the ocean. In reality, these patches are almost entirely made up of tiny bits of plastic, called microplastics. Microplastics can't

"always be seen by the naked eye. Even satellite imagery doesn't show a giant patch of garbage. The microplastics of the Great Pacific Garbage Patch can simply make the water look like a cloudy soup. This soup is intermixed with larger items, such as fishing gear and shoes."

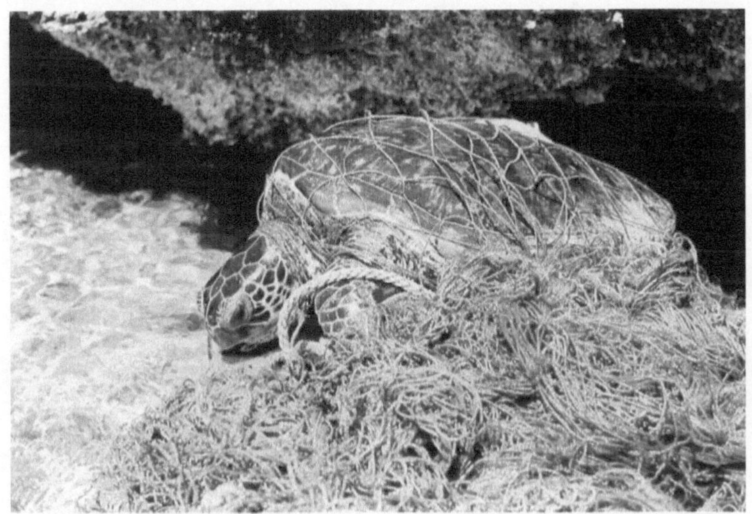

This image makes me feel sick to my stomach.

Sea life should not have to be subjected to the human pollution and waste products that destroy the coral reefs and kill the animals and wild things in the seas and oceans of the earth.

We can do better, and we must, or there won't be any sea life, nor any life at all, to pass on to our children and their descendants.

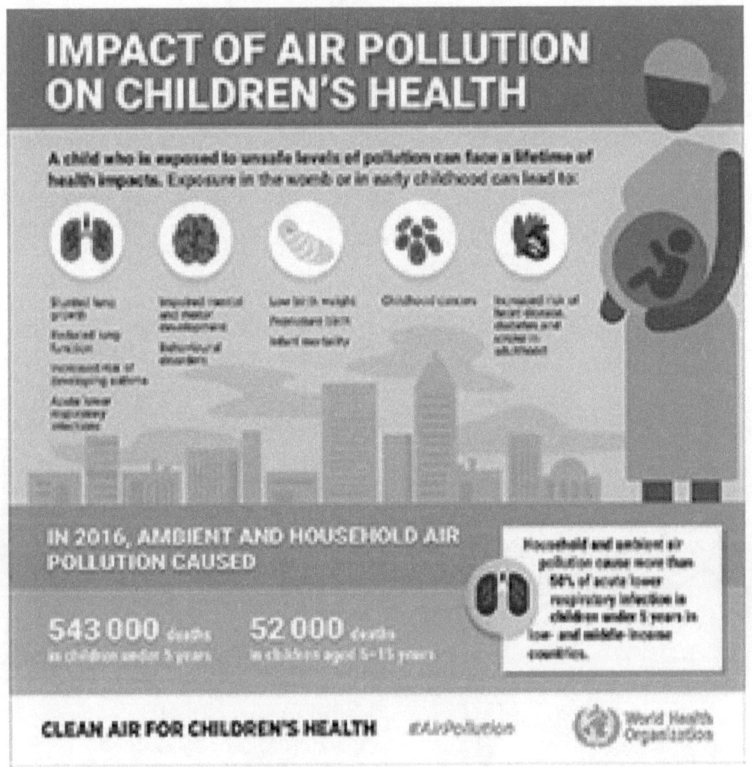

Chapter Five

The Air We Breathe

World Health Organization Facts

Air pollution levels remain dangerously high in many parts of the world. New data from WHO shows that 9 out of 10 people breathe air containing high levels of pollutants.

WHO estimates that around 7 million people die every year from exposure to polluted air.

Ambient air pollution alone caused some 4.2 million deaths in 2016, while household air pollution from cooking with polluting fuels and technologies caused an estimated 3.8 million deaths in the same period.

Every day around 93% of the world's children under the age of 15 years (1.8 billion children) breathe air that is so polluted it puts their health and development at serious risk. Tragically, many of them die: WHO estimates that in 2016, 600,000 children died from acute lower respiratory infections caused by polluted air.

A new WHO report on Air pollution and child health: Prescribing clean air examines the heavy toll of both ambient (outside) and

household air pollution on the health of the world's children, particularly in low- and middle-income countries. The report is being launched on the eve of WHO's first ever Global Conference on Air Pollution and Health.

It reveals that when pregnant women are exposed to polluted air, they are more likely to give birth prematurely, and have small, low birth-weight children. Air pollution also impacts neurodevelopment and cognitive ability and can trigger asthma, and childhood cancer. Children who have been exposed to high levels of air pollution may be at greater risk for chronic diseases such as cardiovascular disease later in life.

"Polluted air is poisoning millions of children and ruining their lives," says Dr Tedros Adhanom Ghebreyesus, WHO Director-General. "This is inexcusable. Every child should be able to breathe clean air so they can grow and fulfil their full potential."

One reason why children are particularly vulnerable to the effects of air pollution is that they breathe more rapidly than adults and so absorb more pollutants.

They also live closer to the ground, where some pollutants reach peak concentrations – at a time when their brains and bodies are still developing.

Newborns and young children are also more susceptible to household air pollution in homes that regularly use polluting fuels and technologies for cooking, heating and lighting

"Air Pollution is stunting our children's brains, affecting their health in more ways than we suspected. But there are many straight-forward ways to reduce emissions of dangerous pollutants," says Dr Maria Neira, Director, Department of Public Health, Environmental and Social Determinants of Health at WHO.

"WHO is supporting implementation of health-wise policy measures like accelerating the switch to clean cooking and heating fuels and technologies, promoting the use of cleaner transport, energy-efficient housing and urban planning. We are preparing the ground for low emission power generation, cleaner, safer industrial technologies and better municipal waste management," she added.

Key findings:

Air pollution affects neurodevelopment, leading to lower cognitive test outcomes, negatively affecting mental and motor development.

Air pollution is damaging children's lung function, even at lower levels of exposures

Globally, 93% of the world's children under 15 years of age are exposed to ambient fine particulate matter (PM2.5) levels above WHO air quality guidelines, which include the 630 million of children under 5 years of age, and 1.8 billion of children under 15 years

In low- and middle-income countries around the world, 98% of all children under 5 are exposed to PM2.5 levels above WHO air quality guidelines. In comparison, in high-income countries, 52% of children under 5 are exposed to levels above WHO air quality guidelines.

More than 40% of the world's population – which includes 1 billion children under 15 - is exposed to high levels of household air pollution from mainly cooking with polluting technologies and fuels.

About 600 '000 deaths in children under 15 years of age were attributed to the joint effects of ambient and household air pollution in 2016.

Together, household air pollution from cooking and ambient (outside) air pollution cause more than 50% of acute lower respiratory infections in children under 5 years of age in low- and middle-income countries.

Air pollution is one of the leading threats to child health, accounting for almost 1 in 10 deaths in children under five years of age.

WHO's First Global Conference on Air Pollution and Health, which opens in Geneva on Tuesday 30 October will provide the opportunity for world leaders; ministers of health, energy, and environment; mayors; heads of intergovernmental organizations; scientists and others to commit to act against this serious health threat, which shortens the lives of around 7 million people each year.

Clean air is vital to runners. I was a long-distance runner until I turned 50 years old. Now I walk for exercise and good health.

When I was running marathons, the air outside made all the difference in the world. I tried not to run where there was car and truck traffic, because the fuel polluted the air and it was hard to breathe.

When I ran in the Colorado Pueblo Marathon, I could really tell the difference in the level of oxygen in the air at a mile above sea level—it was harder to breathe while I was running, and it took a while to train myself to run at that altitude.

Let me tell you a story about my spiritual life that relates to running. I've titled it:

Run and Not Grow Weary

"Those who hope in the LORD will renew their strength. They will soar on wings like eagles; they will run and not grow weary, they will walk and not be faint." (Isaiah 40:31, NIV)

There is no failure for the faithful. Real faith does not grow weary.

When I was running marathons, I never cared about winning a race. The most important thing to me, the thing I was faithful to, and the thing that kept me injury-free year after year, was finishing the race.

That's the only thing that motivated me to keep on running, long after my strength had left me, long past the time when I was exhausted, and long after my muscle's store of glycogen had been depleted.

I was focused on keeping my eye on the goal. The goal was always to finish the race. Remaining faithful to that goal has been the main motivating force of my life. Staying faithful and finishing the race.

Saint Paul the Apostle said it this way, in 2nd Timothy chapter 4, verse 7 (NIV): "I have fought the good fight, I have finished the race, I have kept the faith."

The marathon is a race that is 26.2 miles in length, named in honor of Pheidippides, who was a Greek soldier and a messenger made famous for running from the Battle of Marathon to Athens in Greece. He completed the distance in order to announce to the officials in Athens that they had won the victory.

He, like Paul, finished the race and kept the faith. That was his task. To go the distance and

announce the victory. To this task he was faithful to the very end.

Being faithful to God and family has been the motivating force in my life. When I was baptized at the age of eight, I promised to follow Jesus and be faithful to God throughout my entire life. When I married my wife 55 years ago, I promised to remain faithful to her for my entire life, no exceptions.

I grew up without a father. It was difficult for me at times, but my mother was the one who really made the sacrifice for us three boys. It wasn't easy for her. I love and respect her for all she meant to me, may she rest in peace.

My mother was the one who taught me to be faithful to family and to God. I took her message and example to heart long ago, and I still do.

Since I didn't have a father figure to show me how to be a good father, I learned from my father-in-law Orrice, who was always called "Bud."

I remember the memorial service in Stewartsville, Missouri for my father-in-law Orrice McCord. He was a man of God and a faithful family man. Those were the two most important things in his life, and the things that motivated him throughout his 91 years.

There were many friends and family who spoke at the memorial service, and at the close of the service, the pastor said these words from Matthew 25:21 (KJV), "Well done, thou good and faithful servant: thou hast been faithful over a few things, I will make thee ruler over many things: enter thou into the joy of thy Lord."

Everyone was silent. Everyone had tears in their eyes. I could never begin to match the love and devotion to God and family of that great man, Orrice McCord. He was indeed a faithful servant of our Lord Jesus Christ and a man of great integrity. I think of him each and every day.

I look up to him as my real and spiritual father and mentor. He visits me often in my dreams. I know he is watching over me. May he rest in peace.

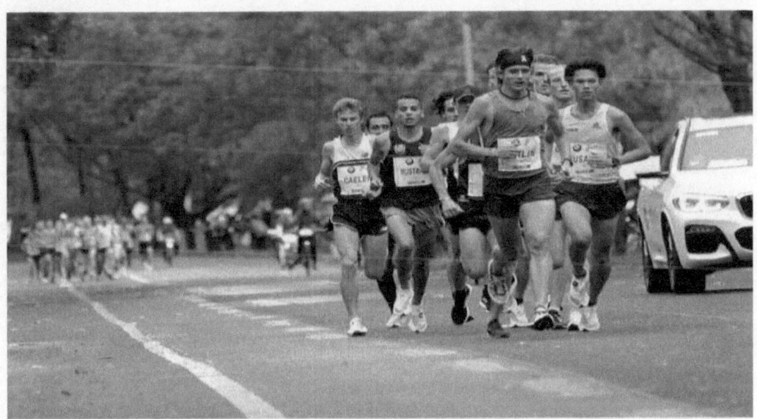

The last and final race of my life is the one I am running now. There are not many miles left for me to run. My goal is to finish the race, and hopefully to have those words spoken at my memorial service,

"Well done, thou good and faithful servant...enter thou into the joy of thy Lord."

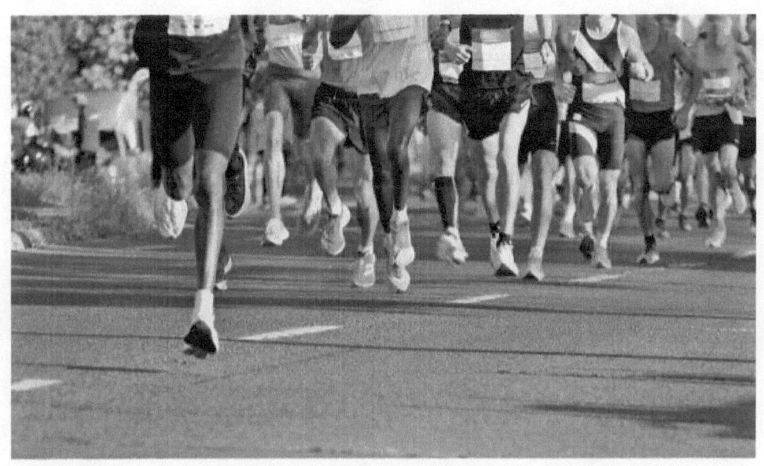

Chapter Six

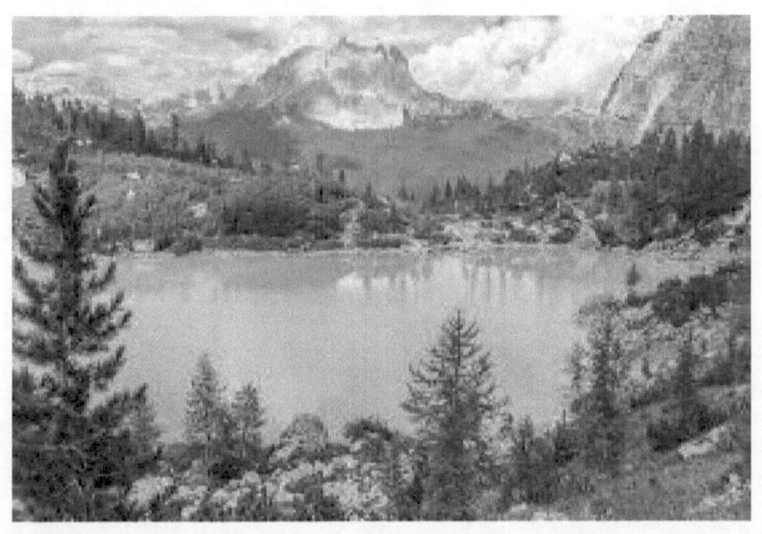

Beautiful Images of Clean Mountain Lakes

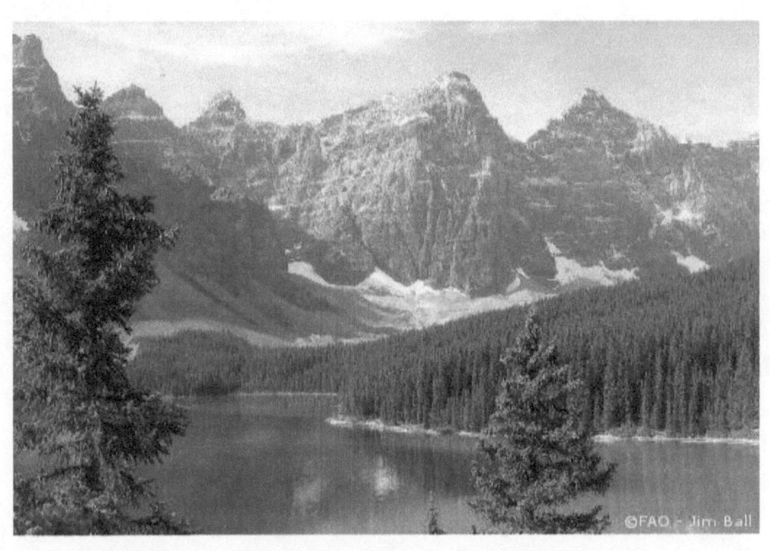

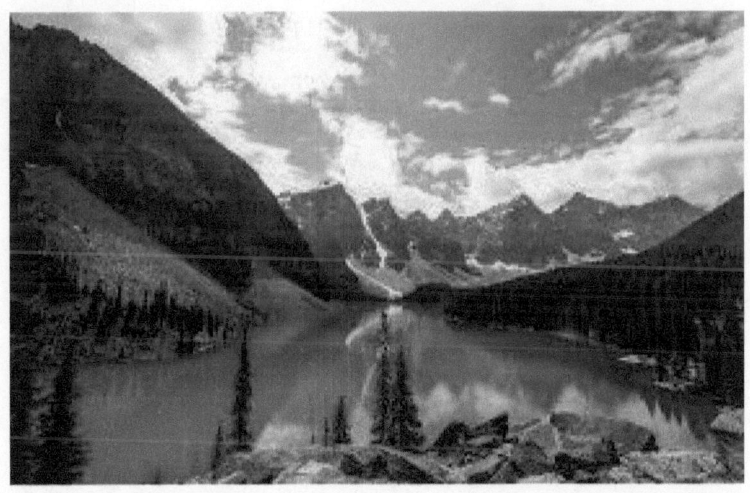

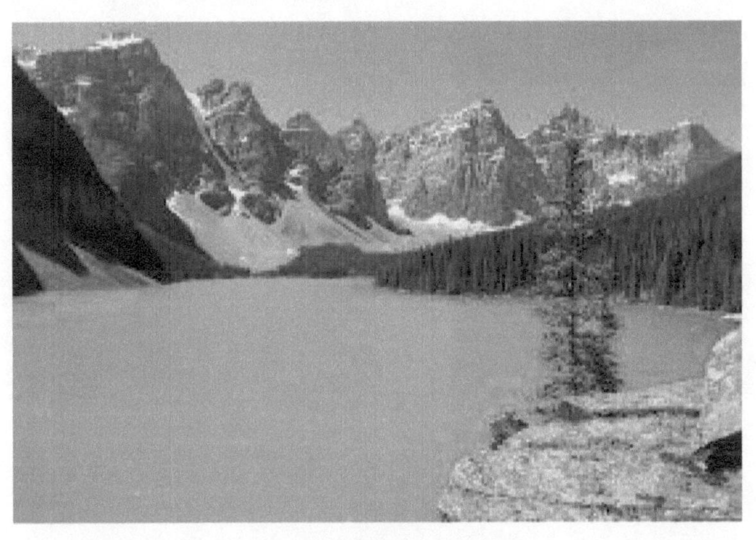

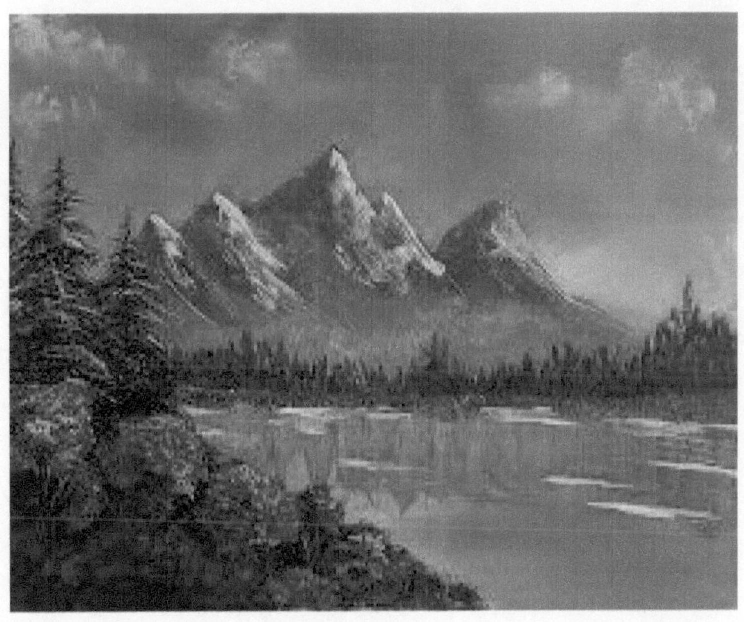

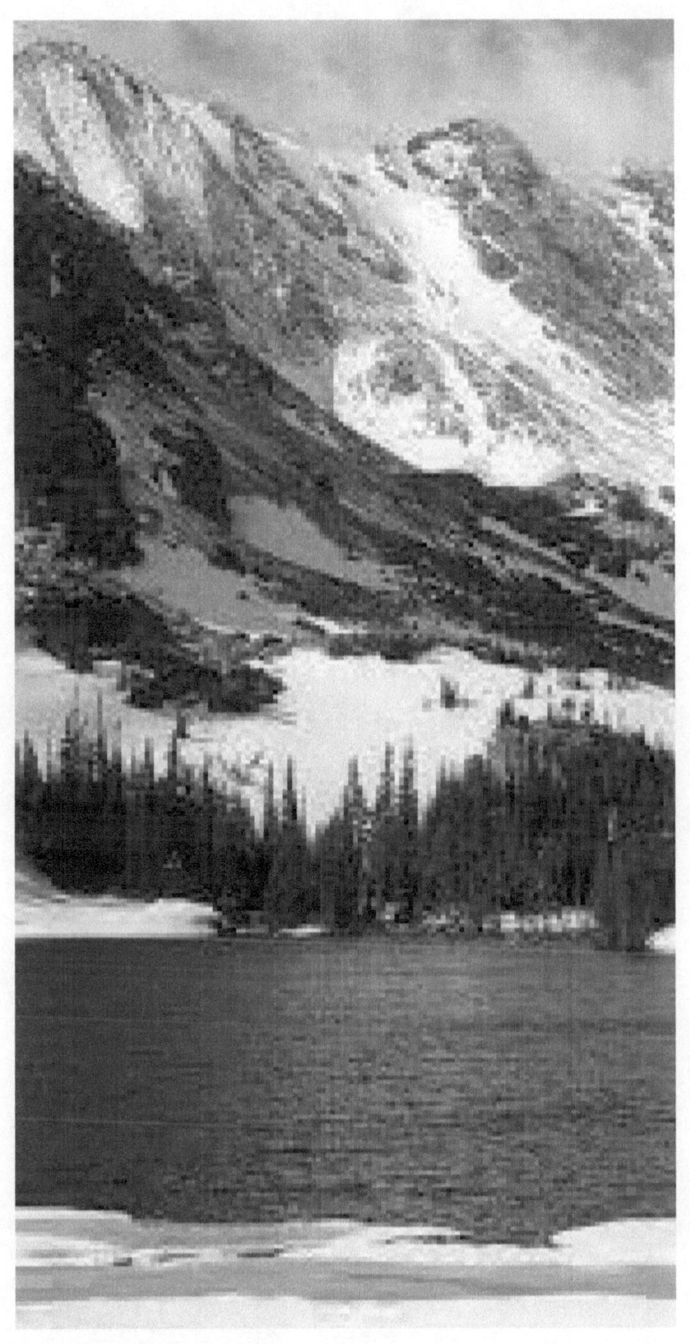

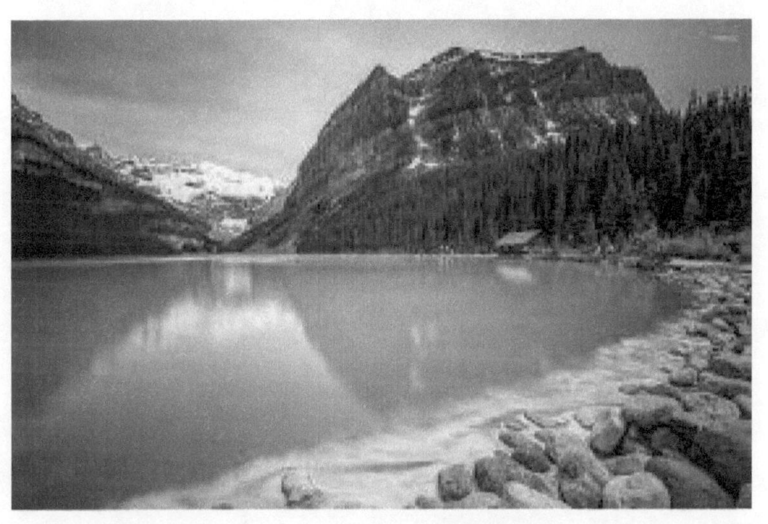

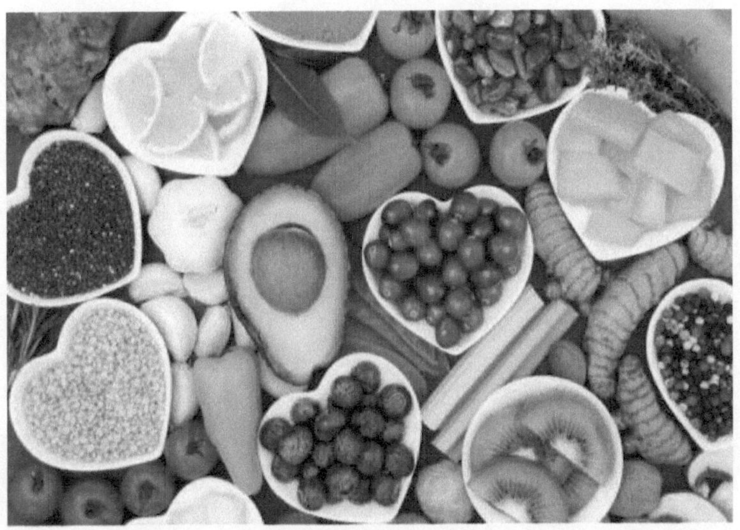

Genesis 1:29: "Behold, I have given you every herb bearing seed, which is upon the face of all the earth, and every tree, in the which is the fruit of a tree yielding seed; to you it shall be for meat."

When God created the earth and the seas, the skies and all the animal kingdom, he made the first man and woman—Adam and Eve.

God provided everything they should need, as written in Genesis 1:29:

"Behold, I have given you every herb bearing seed, which is upon the face of all the earth, and every tree, in the which is the fruit of a tree yielding seed; to you it shall be for meat."

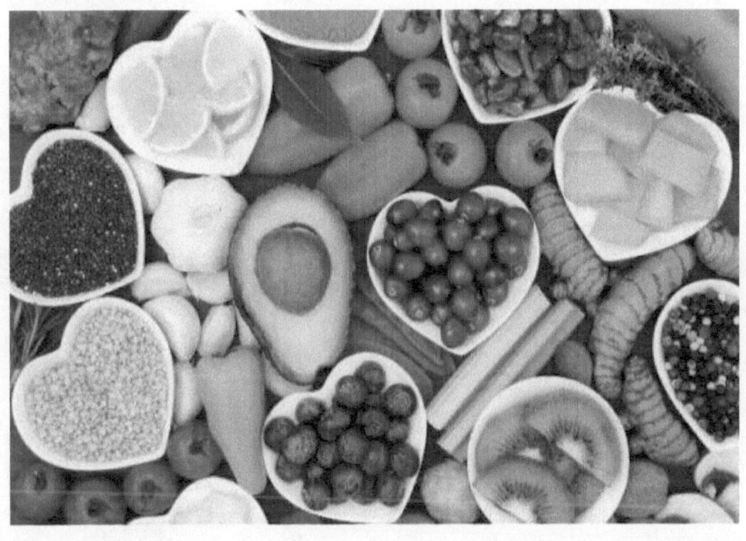

Good, clean, fresh, delicious food from the earth.

Today, most of the food we eat is contaminated, resulting in malnutrition and all manner of disease and disability.

What has happened? Where did we go wrong?

Much of the food we eat contains toxins from fertilizers, pesticides, and fecal matter from corporate farms. Chemicals and industrial waste contaminate our rivers and oceans, finding its way into the food we buy at the grocery stores.

A recent CNN report is alarming, as it points to the poisoning of our most precious resource and hope for the future—our children.

(CNN)Toxic heavy metals damaging to your baby's brain development are likely in the baby food you are feeding your infant, according to a new investigation published Thursday.

Tests of 168 baby foods from major manufacturers in the US found 95% contained lead, 73% contained arsenic, 75% contained cadmium and 32% contained mercury. One fourth of the foods contained all four heavy metals.

One in five baby foods tested had over 10 times the 1-ppb limit of lead endorsed by public health advocates, although experts agree that no level of lead is safe.

The results mimicked a previous study by the Food and Drug Administration that found one or more of the same metals in 33 of 39 types of baby food tested.

(CNN)The US Food and Drug Administration confirmed that PFAS chemicals have made their way into the US food supply. On Monday, the FDA publicly acknowledged the initial findings of the agency's investigation into how the "forever chemicals" have been detected in the foods we eat.

PFAS is a family of nearly 5,000 synthetic chemicals that are extremely persistent in the environment and in our bodies. PFAS is short for perfluoroalky and polyfluoroalkyl substances and includes chemicals known as PFOS, PFOA and GenX, sometimes called forever chemicals. These chemicals all share signature elemental bonds of fluorine and carbon, which are extremely strong and difficult to break down in the environment or in our bodies.

These chemicals can easily migrate into the air, dust, food, soil and water and can accumulate in the body. They've been linked to adverse health impacts including liver damage, thyroid disease, decreased fertility, high cholesterol, obesity, hormone suppression and cancer.

In the body, PFAS chemicals primarily settle into the blood, kidney and liver. A study from 2007 by the US Centers for Disease Control

and Prevention estimated that PFAS chemicals could be detected in the blood of 98% of the US population.

Most of the mercury that contaminates fish comes from household and industrial waste that is incinerated or released during the burning of coal and other fossil fuels. Products containing mercury that are improperly thrown in the garbage or washed down drains end up in landfills, incinerators, or sewage treatment facilities. The mercury then leaches into the ground and water. Once mercury enters the water and soil, it is naturally converted to methyl mercury by bacteria. In water, the bacteria are eaten by plankton and other small creatures, which in turn are eaten by small fish, then larger fish. Mercury doesn't easily leave the body of an organism, so the amount of mercury builds up in species as they go up the food chain in a process called bioaccumulation (PDF).

Pesticides have been linked to a wide range of human health hazards ranging from cancer to endocrine (hormone) disruption and infertility.

Some of the most prevalent forms of cancer that pesticides have been linked with include leukemia, non-Hodgkin's lymphoma, brain, bone, breast, ovarian, prostate, testicular and liver cancer.

According to data from the U.S. Centers for Disease Control and Prevention (CDC), more than 75 percent of the U.S. population has detectable levels of organophosphate pesticides in their urine, with diet being the most likely route of exposure.

Most pesticides directly target both the central nervous system (brain and spinal cord) and the peripheral nervous system (nerves going to the feet, legs, hands, arms and internal organs).

Mounting research has revealed that pesticides, herbicides and fungicides (all chemicals sprayed on fruit and vegetable crops) accumulate in the body and can damage peripheral nerves, brain neurons and organ function.

In February 2009, the Agency for Toxic Substances and Disease Registry published a study that found that children who live in homes where their parents use pesticides are twice as likely to develop brain cancer versus those that live in residences in which no pesticides are used.

Eating organic is one of the best ways to lower your overall pesticide burden. The largest study of its kind found that people who "often or always" ate organic food had about 65 percent lower levels of pesticide residues compared to those who ate the least amount of organic produce.

Research also found that organic produce had, on average, 180 times lower pesticide content than conventional produce.

If you can't afford to buy all of your fruits and vegetables organic, prioritize. You can download the 'Dirty Dozen List' app to your phone. This list is put out every year by the Environmental Working Group (EWG). It will show the fruits and vegetables with the highest to the lowest concentration of pesticides.

It's possible to find produce that is not certified organic that may still have a lower pesticide burden than typical conventional produce depending on the farmer. So if you can't find organic produce, look for a local farmer who has eliminated pesticide use (or uses chemicals only minimally).

There are solutions to the problems of pollution in the earth, the oceans, and the air we breathe. These man-made problems have a man-made remedy, if we only have the will to do what is needed.

Be informed, get involved. There are many good and worthwhile organizations at the forefront of solving these issues. Check them thoroughly before you join, and then volunteer to make a difference.

It's up to you and me to change the future for
our children and our children's
children—they're worth it!

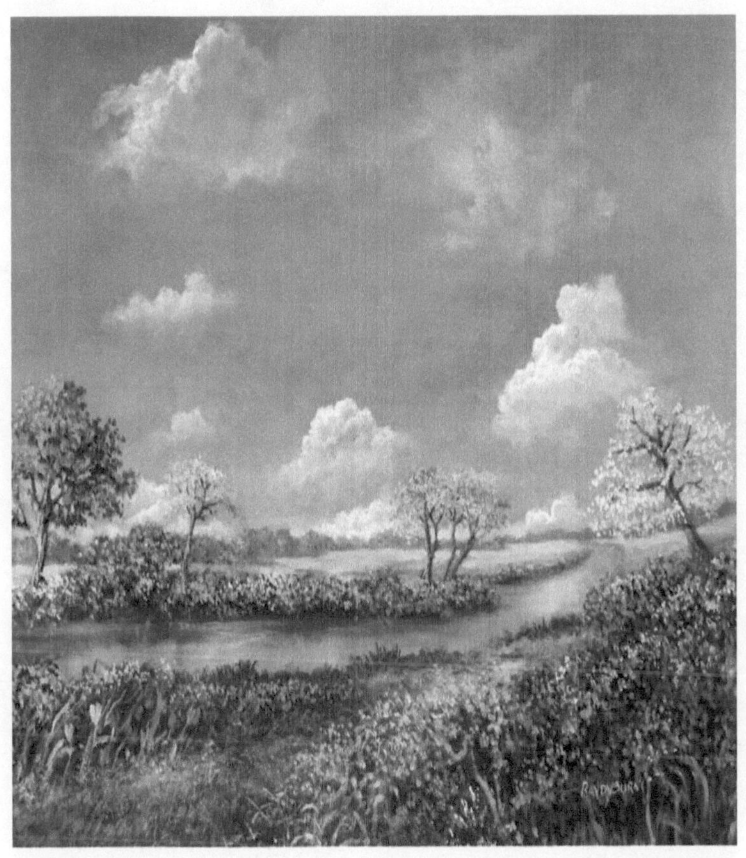

A Prayer of Gratitude and Blessing:

Our Father in Heaven,

Thank you for the gift of Christ and the Holy Spirit, and for all the many gifts and blessings we receive from your gracious bounty. We are so grateful that you sent your son Jesus to live among us, and to show us the way of love. Thank you for his life, his forgiveness, and for his sacrifice on the cross for our salvation. We pray that everyone will come to receive Jesus Christ as the Lord and Savior of their life, and in so doing inherit the Kingdom of Heaven you have prepared for us. May our love increase day by day, and may the peace of Christ live in our hearts, in our homes, and in all the world. In the precious name of Jesus, our Savior and friend. Amen

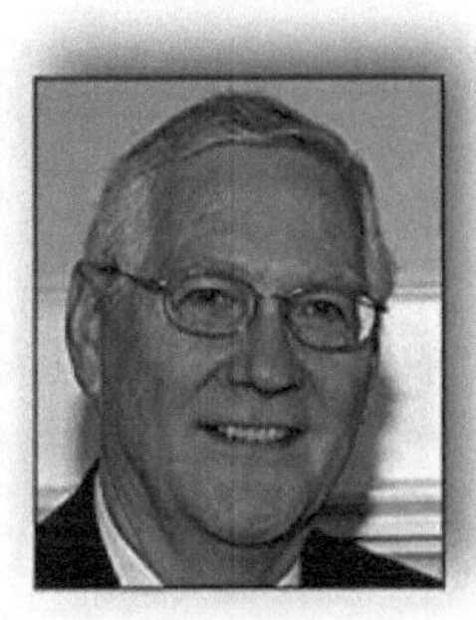

About the Author

Gene Allen Groner is a Christian writer of more than 40 books of faith and inspiration. He also writes articles for the Herald, Daily Bread, and Veterans' Voices magazine. Gene lives in Independence, Missouri with his wife of 55 years, a retired public health nurse. His interests include reading and writing, gardening, and volunteer work in the community. He is listed in Who's Who in Missouri, and is a lifetime member of the National Honor Society in Psychology, Psi Chi. Gene earned both the bachelor's and master's degrees with honors from Park University in Parkville, Missouri. He also attended the University of Hawaii and Saint Paul School of Theology. He and his family are active members of the Colonial Hills congregation in Blue Springs, Missouri.

Write to Gene at geneallengroner@gmail.com

Visit Gene's author page at

https://www.amazon.com/Gene-Allen-Groner/e/B077YTVSJZ

Books by Gene Allen Groner in Print and eBook Available on his author website at https://www.amazon.com/Gene-Allen-Groner/e/B077YTVSJZ

Journey of a Disciple

The Garden of Eden

Native American Prayers Poems and Legends

Native American Horses

Native American Fine Art

Fine Art Paintings

Micah's Fine Art

Fine Art of Sassan Filshoof

Son of the Most High

These Three Remain

The Helper: a Discourse on the Holy Spirit

Hallowed Be Thy Name

Deborah: Prophetess and Warrior

Saint Teresa of Calcutta

From Shepherd to King: the Story of David

The Nature of Angels

A Book of Prayers

Speak To This People: Prophets and Prophecies

For Such a Time as This: the Story of Esther

Prayers and Poems of Christ

In the Beginning

Take Off Your Sandals: the Story of Moses

Silver-Tongued Prophet: the Story of Isaiah

My God is Yahweh: the Story of Elijah

Meditations (in English and Portuguese)

Evangelist Billy Graham

World's Greatest Missionary: the Apostle Paul

Poetry from the Heart

Stairway to Heaven

Full of Grace

Jesus' Hands Are Kind Hands

The Kingdom of Heaven

Women in the Bible

Testify

Revelation

The Cross

The Road to Emmaus

Pentecost

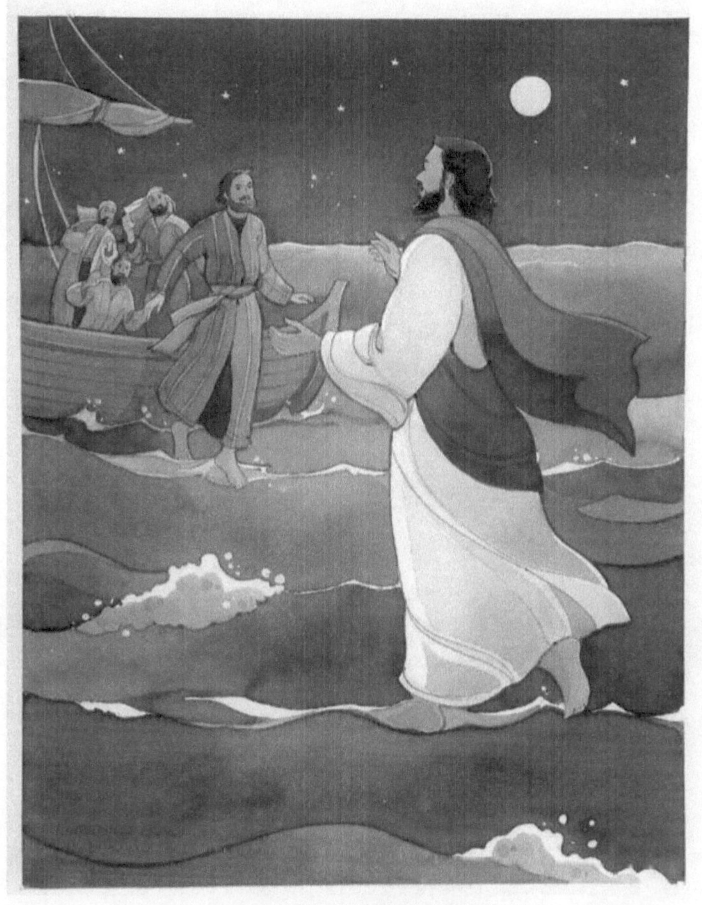

Jesus Loves You

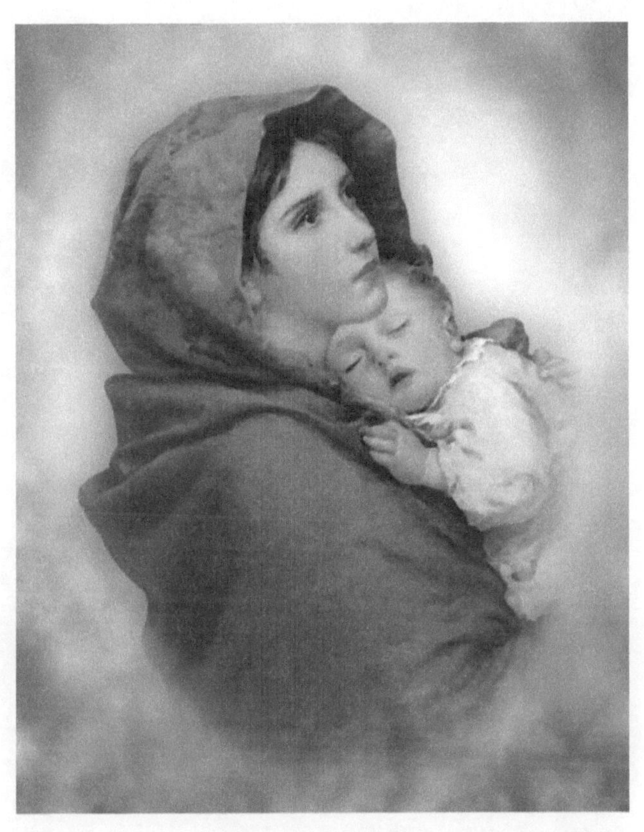